Hair Growth Hacks

Hair Growth Hacks

Hair Growth Hacks

15 Simple Practical Hacks to Stop Hair Loss and Grow Hair Faster Naturally

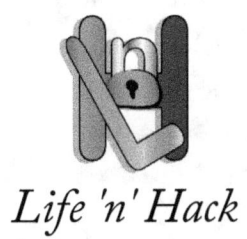

Life 'n' Hack

While attempts have been made to verify the information contained within this publication, neither the author nor the publisher assumes any responsibility for errors, omissions, interpretation or usage of the subject matter herein.

This publication contains the opinions and ideas of its author and is intended for informational purpose only. The author and publisher shall in no event held be liable for any loss or other damages incurred from the usage of this publication.

ISBN 978-1-545-05567-0

Printed in the United States of America

First Edition

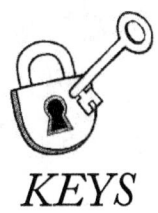

KEYS

INFO INTRO:

The Look Behind Trichology

Hair is your most important accessory. *Why?* You are unique, and a beautiful cut and style that's suited to your facial characteristics can be the simplest thing in the world to magically enhance your appearance more than anything you might ever wear. It's also something that can be changed often, even day to day, like a shirt.

But, after a while, all the processing that goes into it — dyeing, brushing, blow-drying, highlighting, straightening, shampooing, gelling, heat from curling irons and so forth — can take a toll.

Nobody wants to hit 30 and notice patchy gaps on their scalp. So, stop the abuse and start learning more about how to promote healthy and beautiful hair for life.

It may take a little extra effort to pay attention to healthy hair, but consider the rewards:

- Well-kept hair has more volume and shine, contributing to your natural beauty even when you're not wearing makeup.

- Hair is one of those parts of your body that's a barometer for overall good health. There are deeper reasons for hair loss; hormonal problems or pregnancy, for example, could be the reason. But if you're experiencing unusual hair loss, it should be taken seriously as a potential medical issue.

- Well-kept hair is often perceived as a sign of a person who is hygienic. When your hair is beautifully styled, treated and properly moisturized, you send out positive signals about yourself as a well-groomed, self-respecting person who takes care of themselves.

- Lush and beautiful hair can boost your self-esteem and confidence, which in itself will make you more attractive to others, in addition to the already physical enhancement to your looks.

- Good hair reflects higher status. Don't be surprised by how some people would spend a huge fortune on their hair. But continue on: Below, we'll provide you with some cheaper alternatives that will make you look like a million bucks for a fraction of the cost.

Taking care of your hair is a little like taking care of a houseplant. To thrive, a plant needs regular watering, trimming and removal of stray weeds. To keep it looking healthy, you need to dispose of leaves that fall when they die. A bit of care makes it a great addition to your living room décor.

To thrive, your hair also needs applications of water (as you shampoo) and regular trimming to keep it looking its best and to ensure it suits your personal taste and the shape of your face. (And this holds true regardless if you're a woman or a man.)

Before we move on, let's address the obsession some people concerned about their hair have with pills/hair supplements (especially those claiming to be rich in biotin and collagen).

- Biotin helps your body regulate ordinary functions (including hair growth).

- Collagen may be especially beneficial to people who are in their thirties, since it's around that age that our body starts producing less collagen, a process that unfortunately contributes to thinning hair and the beginnings of baldness.

Specialists tend to discourage relying too heavily on these supplements because:

- The beauty benefits of nutrients like biotin have not yet been proven.

- You cannot replace a bad diet with supplements because some features — including a tendency to thinning hair — are given to us naturally.

- A few supplements like Viviscal (a Scandinavian natural hair supplement), have been recommended. But don't put all your hopes on them.

- A better way to ensure great hair is to follow a diet rich in vitamins A and B, zinc and iron. (More will be covered on them later.)

Another popular product on the market for people experiencing hair loss is the FDA-approved Rogaine, also known as minoxidil. It comes in the form of a topical cream or foam and is used by both men and women experiencing a receding hairline or baldness, a condition known as androgenetic alopecia — also known in men as "male pattern baldness." If you're facing this condition, even with the use of Rogaine, growing back their hair will take a long time.

The product claims to show some results around 12 days after use. Although it appears to work for some people, there are drawbacks. For instance:

- To get results, it needs to be applied twice a day on the scalp. This procedure can be a hassle and could lead to the product not being used appropriately.

- It may give you unwanted facial hair. That could be a big "Oops!" for many women out there.

- It can get costly, with a price range of $28 to $30 per item.

Added to this is a scary list of potential side effects like chest pain, fever, chills, sore throat, fainting, and unusual bleeding.

So, unless you suffer from a very severe condition, and you are really desperate for good hair, ask yourself do the benefits outweigh the risks.

If you want to improve the appearance and health of your hair, why not favor natural alternatives, backed up by science.

With that said, let's begin our hacks for beautiful hair.

HACK #1:

Massage Scalp Daily

Massages, in general, are known to help facilitate blood flow in your body, and it benefits hair follicles and the hair itself. When you massage your hair, you are encouraging glowing and fast-growing hair.

On a cultural note, South Asian women, known for growing their hair to great lengths, often massage their hair with oils in order to encourage strong and shiny locks.

Here's how you proceed with a scalp massage:

1. First, decide if you want to massage your hair with no oil or with oil. Both are totally fine, but oils may assist in speeding hair growth, keeping it supple,

improving circulation, or relieving an itchy scalp. Here's a list of ideal oils for scalp massaging:

- Peppermint oil, which will help improve blood circulation.
- Tea tree oil, which will help with an itchy and dry scalp.
- Almond and castor oil, which will help promote hair growth.
- And lastly coconut oil, which you can never go wrong with for anything.

2. Sit down in a calm room where you can take advantage of the soothing effect of the massage. Apply the oil of your choice, if you're using it, to the scalp with the tips of your fingers.

3. Start massaging at the front of your head, beginning at the sides. Use a circular motion, moving slowly from the sides to the center.

4. Continue massaging from the center of your head to the back of your head.

5. Repeat this pattern a total of five times, moving slowly from one spot to another.

6. When done, brush or comb your hair gently.

ASSIGNMENT: Try doing this tonight before going to bed, and in the morning before you start your daily routine. This way you will increase blood flow in your scalp and also promote growth and healthy hair. Don't forget to use your fingertips and opt for an oil if you wish to.

HACK #2:

Bathe Hair with Natural Oils

With constant exposure to air, heat, wind, aggressive hair products and shampoos, your hair can end up being excessively dry and worn out, whether you're a woman or a man. Dry hair breaks easily and starts to look unkempt and unmanageable.

You don't have to pay a fortune for expensive hair moisturizers. Natural oils such as olive oil and coconut oil have been used for generations by communities in the Mediterranean, Asia and Africa to encourage hair strength and growth.

If you've used harsh processes on your hair, like permanents and bleaching, applications of oil can add moisture and suppleness, making the hair less likely to break and easier to style.

Rubbing your hair with natural oils — a "hair bath" — is done after a shampoo:

1. Pat your hair dry with a towel. Do not use a hair dryer.

2. Use 1/4 cup of virgin olive oil or coconut oil.

3. Separate your hair into four sections, from back to front.

4. Rub the oil generously on the hair. Don't apply the oils directly to the scalp. Apply first to the root end of the hair, working your way gradually to the ends.

5. When you are done applying the oil, massage the hair. Then gather your hair together in the middle of

your head, making sure the oil has been spread evenly throughout.

6. Cover your hair with plastic. One of those plastic shower caps you get at a hotel is convenient.

7. Wrap your head with a hot towel and leave it in place for 30 minutes or an hour.

8. When time's up, rinse your hair carefully with cool water and pat dry with a towel.

9. When done, you can use a blow dryer to dry your hair or simply let it dry on its own.

You will find your hair looking and feeling healthier and easier to comb (with less bristled ends).

ASSIGNMENT: If you like the results, use an oil bath once a week to rebuild your hair's natural moisture and prevent breakage. Remember to leave your oil preparation on your hair from 30 minutes and up to an hour.

HACK #3:

Shampoo Properly on Scalp, Not the Ends

One common mistake people make when shampooing is focusing on the wrong part of their hair, that is, the ends, instead of working on the part that most needs to be clean so that it can absorb your after-shampoo treatment: the roots of the hair, near your scalp.

For your hair to grow, the pores on your scalp need to be stimulated. They shouldn't be clogged up with dirt, flakes, etc., so that they can absorb the benefits of nutrients and any other hair "food" you might use to nourish your hair.

This is how a proper shampooing session is done:

1. First, wet your hair under the shower for two minutes. Make sure there's enough water on your hair so that, later on, the shampoo can foam and do its job properly.

2. Next, apply the shampoo evenly (to the front, sides, and back of your head).

3. Start rubbing your head by concentrating on the scalp (away from the water).

4. Focus on the scalp for the next 60 seconds. Don't worry about shampooing the strand all the way down to the tips. When you rinse, the shampoo and water will slide down the hair and automatically take care of cleaning the ends.

5. If you really need to, repeat the process one more time, to make sure that your scalp is totally clean. Applying shampoo no more than twice will ensure a clean scalp and prevent over-drying your hair. Most

people find one application of shampoo is sufficient, despite manufacturer's recommendations to "rinse and repeat."

6. End your shampooing session by rinsing your hair. Use a conditioner if you wish and leave it on the hair for two minutes, to help detangle your hair. If you're using a deep conditioning product, dry your hair with a towel before applying the conditioner and leave it on for 15 minutes, which is supposed to maximize its moisturizing effects.

ASSIGNMENT: Adopt this technique from now on, keeping in mind that you should be concentrating on a clean scalp more than your full length of hair, to prevent breakage and avoid over-drying.

HACK #4:

Don't Overwash Hair

Back in the day, many thought it was best to wash hair as often as possible to keep it clean. If you've been following this regimen for years, you may have noticed that your hair looks flat, dull and weak.

It's recommended to wash less frequently, because water makes the hair swell from the inside which can force the cuticle up. In the long run, too much shampooing leads to weakened and frizzy hair.

So, here's a list of recommendations to help you adjust your hair washing regimen:

1. An ideal hair washing schedule may depend on your hair type:

- For straight hair, 3 times a week.
- For frizzy hair, 2 times a week.
- Coarse hair, once a week.

People with straight hair have more open scalp pores; they often find their hair gets oily and dirty more quickly, so they'll need to shampoo more often compared with other hair types.

2. Remember to concentrate on your scalp when shampooing so your hair stays clean longer.

3. Lastly, finish with your usual hair regimen which might consist of conditioner, drying your hair and applying some kind of hair nutrition.

If you're a daily shampooer, you may find it takes a while for your scalp to adjust, but skipping a day or two during the week will help you abandon an unhealthy habit and avoid the damage that comes with over-washing.

As we move on, you will learn more about different natural (and cheaper) ways to take care of your hair.

ASSIGNMENT: Start experimenting. When you begin routinely skipping a few days a week, you'll soon start noticing the changes in your hair, especially when it comes to volume, strength and appearance.

HACK #5:

Always Finish Rinse with Cool Water

Using hot water while shampooing and rinsing your hair actually helps to dry it out and can leave it brittle.

According to Dr. Sandeep Suttar, of the Hair Transplant and Hair Restoration Centre in Mumbai, hot water strips the protective oils from your hair and should be avoided.

1. From now on, always pre-test the temperature of the water with your hand before putting your head under the shower, and adjust the temperature until it feels cool to lukewarm.

2. Make sure you concentrate on shampooing the scalp rather than the full length of your hair.

3. Finish by letting the cool water run over your whole head so you can thoroughly rinse out all the shampoo.

If you'd rather not have to take your whole shower in cool water, just do the shampoo and rinse first in cool water, with your head under the stream, then turn up the heat and keep your head out of the stream while enjoying that hot, steamy shower.

ASSIGNMENT: Do this and it will help keep your hair healthy and shiny, rather than brittle and dull.

HACK #6:

Use Pre-Shampoo to Avoid Breakage

This is a hack that will help block the damaging effects of some chemicals found in shampoos — the ones that dry out your hair or make them weak, for example, sodium lauryl sulfate and triclosan.

Dermatologists believe that applying a pre-shampoo (or pre-poo) can help you prevent blockages and inflammation that contribute to the thinning of the hair.

So learn to prepare your own pre-shampoo. You can buy products like this from the store, but if you prefer a more natural (and cheaper) alternative, a variety of natural oils and butter can work.

To make it simpler for you, we've come up with a two-in-one alternative that combines natural oils and butter.

Before we start, you should know that you can use ingredients like olive oil, eggs, bananas, shea butter, to name a few. You can experiment for yourself, by mixing the fruits, veggies, or eggs with an oil of your choice. Many natural products can be used to make a mask that will provide a shield against harsh stripping of the hair while you're in the process of shampooing.

For this, we will be using avocado for our pre-shampoo.

1. **The mixture.** Prepare your pre-shampoo by peeling, pitting and mashing a ripe avocado. Mix in three tablespoons of extra-virgin olive oil and two tablespoons of coconut oil, plus 1 tablespoon of castor oil. Mix it all up well to create a uniform mixture.

2. **Heat things up.** Warm your mixture in the microwave for 15 seconds to 20 seconds, just to get it

comfortably warm. Make sure it's not too hot — you don't want to burn your scalp! If you find you've heated it up too much, stir and let it cool for a few seconds.

3. **Work into your hair.** Wet your hair before applying. Divide your hair into four sections and apply the mixture to the hair, section by section, and massage it into the hair. Let it sit for up to 30 minutes. Then shampoo your hair and condition it, the way you usually do.

You can also use an egg pre-shampoo if you feel your hair needs a protein boost. This is especially recommended for people who wear hairstyles that put tight strain on the hair.

1. Prepare your mixture by mixing one well-beaten egg with 1/4 cup of plain yogurt plus three tablespoons of your favorite oil (olive oil, coconut oil or tea tree oil).

2. Apply it to the hair and leave it for 20 to 25 minutes.

<u>Note</u>: Do not warm up this mixture, as microwaving it will cook the egg! And when rinsing, use cold water.

<u>ASSIGNMENT</u>: Try this pre-shampoo method occasionally from now on before washing your hair as usual. Remember to begin with the pre-shampoo, and leave it on your hair for at least half an hour.

HACK #7:

Try Dry Shampoos to Avoid Collateral Damage

Dry shampoos can be found in the form of powders and sprays and are mostly recommended as a handy stopgap between shampoos. But they're also free of the unhealthy sulfates found in many wet shampoos.

Dry shampoos absorb excess dirt and grease in your hair without the use of water. They are ideal when you wish to straighten your hair and don't want to deal with frizzy or curly hair (which most of the time, occurs after a shampoo).

1. If you're trying a dry shampoo for the first time, simply divide your hair into four sections.

2. Then start spraying or sprinkling the dry shampoo into the hair.

3. Massage your hair for one minute.

And that's it! No rinsing required.

After you are done with the "dry cleansing" process, style your hair as you wish.

This practice will help you avoid over-drying or over-processing your hair, which often happens with regular shampoos.

ASSIGNMENT: Starting today, try using dry shampoos every now and then (for instance when you are in a rush and need to wash your hair quickly, or you want to style your hair with more ease). Massage the hair for a minute, and "voila!".

HACK #8:

Substitute Store-Bought Conditioner with Homemade Conditioner

As with shampoos, many conditioners may contain substances that are harmful or irritating, including some that, according to Carly Fraser, owner and founder of Live, Love Fruits, who holds a Bachelor of Science degree in neuroscience, may even be carcinogenic.

Chemicals such as triclosan, potassium glycol, sodium and certain fragrances may be a problem for sensitive individuals, with skin rash, itching, hair breakage and hair loss as some of the possible effects.

Thus, going natural can be beneficial when it comes to your after-shampoo care.

Let's go step by step to make your own natural hair conditioner with one simple ingredient: one fresh egg, composed almost entirely of proteins and fats that will leave your hair nourished and glossy.

1. Beat a raw egg well.

2. Wash your hair: Wet the hair thoroughly with cool water, then apply your shampoo and make sure your hair is clean.

3. Before applying conditioner, pat your hair dry with a towel.

4. Apply half of the beaten egg, leave in for 20 minutes, and then rinse with cool water. Save the rest in a covered container in the refrigerator and save for your next application.

This simple step is all you need to do. Afterward, dry your hair and style as you wish.

ASSIGNMENT: Try this out after shampooing your hair from now on, instead of using harmful chemicals.

HACK #9:

Mix Honey with Existing Conditioner

If you dye your hair over and over again, or you spend most of your summer days swimming in salty or chlorinated water, basking under the sun, and exposing your hair to the drying effects of wind, dust, and pollution, you'll notice that your hair gets more and more damaged, dry, and hard to manage.

Nobody wants to look like a character out of the "Trolls" movie, right?

Here's another sweet trick for boosting the efficacy of your favorite conditioner. Add honey, honey! Here's how to do it:

1. Measure out 1/2 cup of your favorite conditioner.

2. Mix in two or three tablespoons of 100% organic raw honey. Honey is known to be a natural humectant, which helps to retain moisture. It is also full of antioxidants and nutrients that feed hair follicles and encourage hair growth as well.

3. Add some water — about 1/4 cup — to this preparation, which will diminish the stickiness.

4. Shake well and distribute on your hair after you've shampooed it.

5. Leave it in for 30 minutes and then rinse thoroughly.

6. Finish by drying your hair and styling as you wish.

You will find yourself with hair with much more radiant and volume, and a healthier appearance.

<u>ASSIGNMENT</u>: If you decide you like the effect of this idea, you can make it easy on yourself by preparing the solution in advance, adding diluted honey into the bottle with your conditioner. You should see a difference from the very first application.

HACK #10:

Apply Lemon for Dull Hair Problems

This next hair miracle natural remedy might come as a big surprise.

It seems lemon has some good hair benefits such as helping to fight dandruff, relieving an itchy scalp, acting as a natural hair straightener, and even encouraging hair growth.

Also, in some African countries, lemon juice is used by women to alleviate hair loss problem, particularly seen around the hairline, caused by a habit of constantly braiding their hair a little bit too tight (we will come to this in another hack), or to counter hair loss after pregnancy.

Lemons contain a lot of vitamin C, which may give hair the natural boost it needs.

The easy recipe for fighting dull hair and improving its overall appearance is to apply one tablespoon of lemon juice onto hair (after shampooing and thorough rinsing). Then use a towel to dry excessive liquid and style your hair as usual.

- **For an itchy scalp**: Mix a few drops of lemon juice with your shampoo and conditioner (add to the bottles). Use both products regularly and start seeing some improvement.

- **For an oily scalp**: If you find yourself with too much sebum on your scalp, apply lemon juice to the hair to help absorb the excess.

- **For dandruff**: If you've spent most of your life avoiding wearing dark clothes because it makes those dry flakes so obvious, try the following: Mix some lemon juice (about 4 tablespoons) with water. Leave in for about 10 minutes, then rinse the hair.

- **To help straighten your hair:** Mix 1/4 cup of lemon juice and 1 cup of coconut oil. Spread evenly on hair and you've got yourself a natural hair straightener.

ASSIGNMENT: Try one of these lemon recipes for your hair this week and see some overnight results, with cleaner and straighter hair.

HACK #11:

Go for Homemade Hair Sun Treatment

According to Dr. Sandeep Suttar again, honey, eggs and olive oil mixed together help replenish the keratin protein bonds in your hair; keratin is a protective protein.

Here's how:

1. Mix 1/2 cup of honey with 2 tablespoons of olive oil and 2 tablespoons of well-beaten egg yolk.

2. Mix well, until you the mix is smooth and homogenized.

3. After washing your hair, separate hair into four sections and carefully apply the mixture evenly on your hair, section by section.

4. Leave in for 20 minutes and rinse with lukewarm (not hot) water.

Let the hair dry and style as wished. This is excellent if you spend a lot of time under the sun, and will add a protective shield to your hair.

ASSIGNMENT: Now, it's your turn to get to work. Mix half a cup of honey with 2 tablespoons of olive oil and egg yolk. Use this treatment every time you wash your hair on a hot sunny day.

HACK #12:

Tight Hairdos and Extensions Maintenance

Trying out different hairstyles is a great way to express your creativity and individuality.

- Take, for example, braids of all kinds have been used throughout different cultures as a favorite way to keep hair tidy and fashionable. Some even use artificial hair extensions to add lushness to the look. But when braids are routinely done too tight, the practice can result over time in hair loss, in dandruff (because you can't wash your hair with long-term braids), and a very itchy scalp. And that is not all; after undoing the braids, you may find that your hair has become dry and brittle, making it difficult to detangle.

The best alternative would be to:

1. Treat your hair before you decide to use any sort of extensions.

2. Go for a hairstyle that will prevent your hair from being damaged from being done too tightly, or buying a wig that can be removed any time you need to wash your hair and treat it.

3. Moisturize your scalp and hair with a nourishing natural treatment such as shea butter or coconut oil:

- Melt 1/4 cup of natural shea butter or coconut oil.

- Apply on the hair, massage well, so that it gets on the scalp and hair, and leave for 30 minutes.

- After 30 minutes, rinse with cool water, and dry. Your hair will feel less dry, stronger and easy to comb whenever you decide to remove a tight hairdo.

This method was used by women in West Africa, who will apply a generous amount of shea butter before creating an exotic hairstyle that they plan to keep in place for a while. This helps preserve the hair.

4. One last thing is to avoid tying your hair with elastic. Use hair accessories made out of fabric, silk, etc., which will be much easier on the hair fibers.

ASSIGNMENT: From now on, avoid elastics, tight hairdos and always treat your hair before you decide to wear extensions, and make sure any tied hairstyles are not too tight (to prevent hair loss).

HACK #13:

Upgrade Combs/Brushes and Combing/Brushing Techniques

Have you ever thought that maybe the reason combing or brushing your hair becomes a static-y disaster is because you're using the wrong hair implement?

Most people don't know better, so they buy cheap tools for this job, such as plastic combs and brushes with plastic bristles. The danger with these is that they are rough on the scalp, produce heat because they produce static, and can even weaken the hair follicles.

On the other hand, more natural options, such as wooden combs and brushes with boar bristles, may cost a little more, but they will make styling your hair more pleasant and help keep your hair in top condition. Wooden combs and brushes with boar bristles:

- Help distribute natural oils produced by your scalp evenly on the scalp and through your hair, keeping it protected, soft and lustrous.

- Help remove loose hair and clean out dust and lint.

- Are easier on your hair, leaving it softer and polished.

With the best brushing/combing tool you should apply the appropriate brushing/combing approach:

1. Always start by brushing the ends first, in order to gently remove tangles.

2. Follow by taking long strokes from the roots of the hair to the ends.

3. Use Grandma's technique of counting while you brush your hair. Grandma usually counted to 100, but she didn't have all the moisturizers and hair conditioning tips we've shown you today, so you can keep it to 30.

4. One last pointer to keep in mind during the day. If you find yourself needing to "fix your hair" now and then, try using your fingers to straighten it out rather than repeated combing. This will help you avoid losing hair and damaging it with excessive tugging.

ASSIGNMENT: If you are not a person who likes to brush or comb your hair very much, try it this time by buying a wooden comb or a brush with boar bristles. Using the appropriate combing/brushing technique by detangling the tips first, then working on the body. Adopt a habit of fixing your hair every now and then with your fingers.

HACK #14:

Trim Hair Regularly

This is one obvious means of keeping your hair in great condition and clearly improving its appearance.

Hair can grow by a few inches in four months, and when it's not properly moisturized or regularly treated, it has a tendency to become dry, especially at the tips, where breakage produces evenness and a generally unhealthy look. Untrimmed hair, especially with a lot of split ends, also tends to snarl and get knotted more easily when you find yourself in a high wind!

So, here are some simple steps to follow if you want to give yourself a micro-trim every now and then, between professional haircuts:

1. After washing and styling (your hair is wet and more manageable for trimming purposes), separate your hair into sections.

2. Checking in a mirror, measure the length of the hair, and verify if it's even (from one side to another).

3. Pinch a hair bunch 1 inch to the end and cut off half an inch. Carry on the same way with the rest of your head, methodically making sure you cut half an inch to the end of the hair and with the same amount of hair each time.

4. Routine trims will help promote healthier hair (not dry and split ends) and obviously add the look of more volume to your hair.

ASSIGNMENT: You don't need to spend a fortune on a fancy salon; you can trim your own hair. However, if you insist, just get a good stylist or barber who understands your type of hair and what you'd like, and can reproduce your preferred cut every time you visit — say about every six weeks or so.

HACK #15:

Change Diet to Promote Healthy Hair "from the Inside"

"You are what you eat," as they say, and that includes your hair. Even though hair, in a sense, is dead beyond the roots, good nutrition is a huge advantage in building healthy, beautiful hair that continues to look good for months as it grows longer.

According to health and lifestyle writer Catherine Roberts, the following raw fruits and vegetables (and nuts) should be a major part of your diet:

- **Swiss chard**: It is a natural source of biotin, which helps regulate your body and your hair.

- **Salmon/sardines/trout/flaxseeds**: Because they are rich in Omega 3 fatty acids, they help balance the oils in your body, and reduce flakiness as well as itchiness issues.

- **Carrots**: High in vitamin A, a nutrient responsible for cell growth.

- **Chicken/eggs**: Both are rich in protein and can help prevent hair loss. You should eat them as much as you can.

- **Brazil nuts**: These are packed with selenium, a mineral that helps with body functions such as growth and glow of your hair.

- **Spinach/citrus fruits/broccoli/peppers/tomatoes**: They are all a great source of vitamin C, which helps regulate the oil production on your scalp. These foods are good if you have oily hair.

- And of course, **water** for natural hydration and helping getting rid of toxins. Drink up to 10 glasses of water every day.

ASSIGNMENT: This will be your exercise right now: grab a pen and a piece of paper and start putting a list together with the veggies and fruits listed above, and slowly insert them in your diet for better-looking hair.

INFO UNLOCKED:

The Out-of-Salon Look Revealed

Whether you are a woman or man, young or old, your hair means a lot. Like your face, it's a huge component of how you present yourself to the world, and a big reflection of your own unique personality.

Whether we keep it long or short, it's important that your hair always looks shiny, healthy and well-kept. Beautiful hair will leave a positive impression and impact those around you.

The steps to better hair can be easy and accessible, even if you can't afford pricey salons and designer products. You can grab some lemons and eggs from your kitchen and come up with excellent do-it-yourself homemade remedies and treatments.

And while you're in the kitchen, grab some natural oils like olive oil and coconut oil, items you probably use every day already. They can give you great results without worries about harmful chemicals with unknown effects on your body.

Finally, learn to eat better: Eat lots of fresh and healthy foods rich in zinc, selenium, protein and vitamin C. They will help you absorb excessive sebum secretion, fight hair loss, and moisturize your hair naturally.

Start today on implementing some of these fun and easy hacks. Onward now to beautiful healthy hair!

Hair Growth Hacks